Depression Help

How To Cure Depression Naturally and Help Others To Do the Same

Disclaimer

This book contains content generated by us. The content in this book is provided for general information only. It is not intended to amount to advice on which you should rely. In particular, this information is not a substitute for professional medical care by a qualified doctor or other healthcare professional. If you are not a healthcare professional then you should ALWAYS check with your doctor if you have any concerns about your condition or treatment and before taking, or refraining from, any action on the basis of the content on our book. If you are a healthcare professional then this information (including any professional reference material) is intended to support, not replace, your own knowledge, experience and judgement.

Copyright

necessary, legal or professional, a practiced individual in the profession should be ordered.

Table of Contents

Introduction

„Progress is impossible without change, and those who cannot change their minds cannot change anything."

- George Bernard Shaw

The problem in the modern culture - we are never taught how to listen to our emotions and understand their messages for us. We see our emotions as an antagonists to our happiness rather than an intrinsic part of our abundance and well-being. When our emotions are "negative", we seek to drown them out in alcohol, video games, drugs, shopping, or any other means of escape.

When people don't listen to their emotions, they have no choice but to *scream* louder. Instead of a gentle whisper that we are moving in the wrong direction, they start waking us at night and constantly remind about themselves. Usually, they overwhelm us at seemingly random or inappropriate moments. Depression means there is one or more emotions trying to get their **resourceful** message to us, but we are **scared** of listening.

We are trying to drown those messages out, so now the emotions are constantly with us, waiting for us to listen, shouting louder and louder until our whole organism can do nothing but hear the screams.

Chapter 1.

The First Step

"Your depression is connected to your insolence and refusal to praise."

- Rumi

This chapter is a must read if You want to help someone

What actually is depression? In this section I hope to give you a brand new and **healthy** perspective regarding this topic and a brief technique that will give you more self-knowledge and insight, along with an instant feeling of relief.

One of the myths propagated about depression is that you have to suffer for a long time, or recover then relapse. This is totally not true. **Shift might happen in an instant** and lasting recovery is far more common than relapse.

Dear reader, don't get me wrong, but our doctors, counselors and nurses do a great job. If your (or your friends') depression has lasted for a long time or is now causing you physical illness or thoughts of harming yourself or anyone else you should definitely seek help of a health practitioner.

You must use your emotions to conquer this challenge. I know it certainly doesn't feel like this at the moment as the sadness and despair can feel overwhelming, although, once you understand that these emotions have a positive message, your life will **instantly change** and you'll even begin breathing a deep sigh of relief.

Can depression be resourceful? According to evolutionary psychology, depression has evolved to help us to re-assess our life, our direction, and to start shutting down our whole organism as we need time to stop, recover, re-evaluate our lives and **achieve greatness.**

As you start to understand your emotions better, you will feel more grounded and you'll start to **trust yourself** and your **inner wisdom**. We can now begin to see all of our emotions, including depression, as helpful and positive guidance from our unconscious mind, alerting us that we may be moving in the wrong direction and to adjust our course.

There's nothing to lose, but everything to gain! By buying this manuscript, you've taken your first step toward a happier life.

Summary of Previous Chapter

1. Shift might happen in an instant.

2. Your emotions to conquer this challenge.

3. Start to trust yourself and your inner wisdom.

4. Don't forget about Emotional Intelligence (EQ).

5. Myth - It's very slow process of recovering from depression.

6. Depression might be resourceful.

Chapter 2.

How to Spot Your Partner's Depression

„When we are no longer able to change a situation - we are challenged to change ourselves."

- Viktor E.Frankl

It's time we took a look at some of the causes and symptoms of depression. This chapter is specifically designed to give you some indication if you or **your loved ones** are truly suffering from depression, and some possible triggers for depression. This is not uncommon problem – millions on people are dealing with depression everyday! It's actually considered as one of the **most common** mental illnesses. In my opinion, depression is part of the **wisdom inside you** trying to guide, heal you and improve your life. Everyone has the tendency to feel sad from time to time. However, depressed people face more challenges than normal sadness. In fact, most of them can feel hopeless. They feel like they're living in a dark tunnel and they have no idea how to get out of this situation. Meditation could start to give you some self-awareness and mental clarity. Believe me, all these negative thoughts inside your head are false.

Here I will list the common symptoms of depression:

1. Weight Gain or Weight Loss

One of the visible signs of depression is a sudden weight change. You could either lose weight or gain weight. Please be aware of your eating habits, think about changing your meal-plan. Binge-eating/overeating is one of the most popular, but **unhealthy** ways of dealing with depression.

2. Feelings of sadness, crying

We all get sad from time to time, it's nothing special. Although, people with depression are always sad and negative towards others. If you're constantly crying, you are most likely suffering from depression. Don't forget that mood-changes are also sign of a depression.

3. Isolation

If you've been staying the house for days because of your bad mood, then you may be suffering from depression. Depressed people feel disconnected, including their family and friends. For this reason, they tend to isolate themselves from other people. Seeing others might make them more depressed.

4. Hopelessness

If you or people you care about are suffering from depression, you will find it hard to see past your current situation. You will have a hard time believing that your current situation and current circumstances will get better.

5. Pessimism

People with depression have a lot of negative thoughts. If you find it challenging to expect happiness, then you are most likely suffering from depression, anxiety and/or low self-esteem.

6. Low self-esteem

Studies show that people who have low self-esteem are more likely to suffer from depression.

7. Traumatic experiences

Traumatic experiences such as an accident, rape and physical or mental abuse can often lead to depression.

8. Job loss or unemployment

Studies show that most people who are unemployed are susceptible to depression. Also, if you are currently in debt, then you are **more** likely to feel depressed.

9. Serious illness

According to studies, people who have serious illness such as cancer are susceptible to depression. Depression is, in fact, one of the symptoms of other serious diseases.

10. Loss of interest in fun things

People who are depressed often lose interest in activities they used to enjoy doing. When you are depressed, you will not feel excited over the thought of going anywhere outside your house. In fact, you may pass on the opportunity.

11. Low libido / lack of sexual desire or intimacy

Low libido, low will to sex is also one of the most common symptom of depression / anxiety.

12. Lack of goals and dreams

If you are depressed, you will feel a strong sense of hopelessness. As a result, you will not have any dreams or goals. When you are depressed, you will not bother to set goals. You will not even bother to dream of better days ahead.

13. Frequent thoughts of suicide

When you are depressed, you hate this world and your circumstances. You often think about ending your own life. If that's the case, you need to seek a professional help!

14. Drugs

Based on studies, around thirty percent of people who suffer from substance abuse and drug addiction also suffer from depression.

15. Genetics.

If your parents are often depressed, you are more likely to suffer from this at some point in your life. Many studies show that depression can be inherited.

Death of a loved one Sadness caused by the death of a loved one may eventually lead to depression. It is normal to feel sad when you lose a loved one. However, if your sadness is already crippling you, then it is time to ask for help.

16. Abuse and trauma.

Mental, sexual and physical abuse during childhood could lead to depression later in life. The pain caused by past traumatic events can resurface during adulthood.

I include all of these symptoms and possible causes to give a basic presentation of the facts of depression. One of the worst feelings during depression is the feeling that you will never **rise**. Don't worry, friend – **you will**. No feeling or thought lasts forever. If you did the self-awareness exercise in previous chapter you will realize that your mind is very complex and **always** busy! It will move on from the state of depression, simply because it's not what your mind and body wants. You won't stay put for long. This book is designed to just nudge you, to get you unstuck a little quicker than would happen anyway. If you take one thing away from this book, it can be this: this too will pass. Your depression will evade even if you did very little about it. You're changing constantly. You cannot stay depressed for long. The season changes from winter to spring, the clouds pass over the sun, the new seed grows in the earth. You are experiencing very important moment of change of your life. **Depression is essential for growth!**

Summary of Previous Chapter

You learned about symptoms of depression in the previous chapter, let's repeat them:

1. Weight Gain or Weight Loss

2. Feelings of sadness, crying

3. Isolation

4. Hopelessness

5. Pessimism

6. Low self-esteem

7. Traumatic experiences

8. Job loss or unemployment

9. Serious illness

10. Loss of interest in fun things

11. Low libido / lack of sexual desire or intimacy

12. Lack of goals and dreams

13. Frequent thoughts of suicide

14. Drugs

15. Genetics.

16. Abuse and trauma.

Chapter 3.

How can you support your depressed partner, friend, relative

„Sometimes it's the smallest decisions that can change your life forever."

Keri Russell

It's time to discuss some lesser known ways of conquering depression, feeling happiness and understanding ourselves on more deeper level. During depression we may start getting pessimistic, cynical and dosed down and start taking everything in life extremely seriously. I encourage you to stay open-minded to these ideas and try one today. There's nothing to lose.

Here are some suggestions on how you can help your sick partner and support him:

First and foremost, **inform yourself** about the depression. The more you know about depression, the sooner you can classify the symptoms and behaviors of your partner and support him. Thankfully, you've already taken the first step towards it - **by buying this book.**

Very important note: do not take your partner everything from, but not overwhelm him/her also. It is important for him/her that he has the experience to get himself settled a bit.

Playfulness

Taking life and circumstances too seriously can very quickly lead to depression. We can view life as a great blessing, a great curse, or anything in between. Maybe we aren't meant to take everything so seriously. Perhaps simply viewing our roles, be they bus driver, police officer, business owner, mother, boyfriend, uncle, teacher as just games to be played will free us from a great deal of stress and depression over our life conditions. For sure, we are to play these games as best we can, so let's play them full out. But let's still treat them as a game, and perhaps rather than finding them stressful, we can see them as an expression of our joy and creativity as we play and take them in good humor.

Emotional Intelligence

There is a belief in the self improvement industry today that "thoughts are things" and we must strive to keep our thoughts as positive as possible in order to "attract" only positive things into our lives. How exhausting! If you've spent even one minute in meditation, you'll realize that the effort to keep all our thoughts on one track is practically impossible! Now, it is true that thoughts can influence our lives, but only if two conditions are in place. Firstly, we must take the thought seriously and believe that it can influence our life. Secondly, we must act on the thought. So, if we don't take our thinking too seriously and if we don't act on our thoughts, they have absolutely no power whatsoever. They are simply clouds floating in the sky of our consciousness. So, during this temporary feeling of depression, don't take your thoughts too seriously. Don't waste time trying too hard to change your thoughts or fight them or struggle with them or analyze them. Thoughts are just dreams, a monkey jumping from branch to branch, an over-enthusiastic puppy pulling at the leash of our consciousness. Just watch your thoughts. Create a little distance between you and your thinking. Learn to laugh at your thoughts and enjoy your mind jumping around! It can't harm you! Once you see your thoughts for what they are, you'll notice something strange. Your thoughts will slow down and give you more peace and space. When your thoughts slow down, you will feel more "present", whole, healthy and at ease. When our thoughts slow down, our mind recharges and rests, it heals and creates space for insight and understanding. You will be more intelligent and more capable.

Use your creativity and imagination

Although your thoughts are not real, and you shouldn't take them seriously or let them panic you, they can create some real effects in your body. We can use that to our advantage! Remember, if you are depressed, you probably have a greater imagination and creative capacity than most people! As soon as you wake up in the morning, begin imagining that today will be a totally different day, that today something beautiful and incredible is on its way to you, that a brand new opportunity will be revealed, or that something of tremendous value will be discovered. Get a feeling of bubbling excitement and radiant joy. Take as long as you need. Get up in that feeling and stay open to any opportunity that comes your way in that day.

At any point in the day, again get that feeling back, imagine the very best things happening to you and you waving goodbye to depression as you begin enjoying yourself so much that you don't even know how, but your life is getting better and better as you feel so much better inside now.

Acceptance

This one is very counter-intuitive. When we feel depression, we try to do everything we can to fight it, drown it out and shake it off. However, it can often feel like the more we try, the more it persists, further spiraling us into depression. Only by acceptance can change happen though. Rather than fighting with yourself you could just accept that right now, you are depressed.

The reason this works so well is because of the nature of our emotions as discussed in chapter one. Our emotions need our acceptance in order to deliver their message and leave us in peace. This means feeling them, understanding them and accepting them. They are a part of you. Close yourself to your emotions and you close yourself to all of the joy in life.

Love is the cure

Usually, if the flow of joy and happiness has stopped in our life, it is because the flow of love has stopped. Perhaps the job you loved has been lost, or the family member you loved, or the partner, or the creative passion. If this is the case, I and everyone else understands what you're going through. It truly is a terrible experience and one that we must all go through. Once the flow of love is cut however, the flow of our joy can get cut with it. We need to give our love once again in order to feel the joy flow in our lives. Please don't wait for someone to give you love first. This is very miserly. The way we get love is by giving love. This doesn't mean that that special someone we pine over will love us back, that's their prerogative, but it does mean that if we are a more loving person, we are generally more loved in return. It also means that we can find anything to give our love to. It could be a child, a parent, a tree, a rock, a cloud, a partner, ourselves, a pet, a plant, a hobby. Once you start giving your love again, you'll realize a part of you melts and your joy can start to flow again. Once you begin feeling that love being returned to you (give it time) you'll feel overjoyed!

Express gratitude

Our depression causes our focus to narrow down and lock in on all the bad conditions of our life. This is a good thing. We know now that it causes us to think about these conditions because there is an important message for us, a lesson we need to learn, a new wisdom to digest. However, if we have been depressed for a long time, we may become habituated to looking at all that is wrong with our life. We need to counter that habit.

We can start doing this by keeping a list of all the things that are right with our life. We can do this in whatever way we enjoy, we could write a list, make a spreadsheet, keep a journal, kneel and pray, tell them to a friend or just remember them in our head.

As you think about them, really imagine them and experience them in your mind. Feel the emotion of gratitude. You may struggle at the moment to think of anything you can be grateful for. This is your narrowed focus speaking, not the truth! Maybe you and your partner have broken up, but you can still be grateful for your smoking hot body! Perhaps you have been diagnosed with an illness but can be grateful that this has made you realize you need to be present in every moment and give all of your love so that you create a legacy of love and joy for your family and friends. Or maybe you hate your job and can't see a way out but are grateful for the amazing brain you are blessed with. Or the fact that billions of years of ordered creation or random chaos even lead to you having a life at all.

Nothing stands still

The nature of life is flux. Everything is constantly **changing**. This includes all of the conditions of your life, your health, your loved ones, your relationships, your career and your depression. Your depression will change, your feelings will change. Can you honestly say that you are depressed 24 hours a day? There will be times when you sleep, or forget you are depressed and laugh at that sitcom on TV, or feel sad, then angry, then at peace, then tired, then relatively happy. Once you really understand that everything in life changes, you may come to a new level of wisdom. I don't know what that will be for you. For some people, once they realize that everything in life changes, they understand they don't need to keep grasping, they can let go, they don't need to hang on to conditions or prevent them from changing, and all they really can do is give their loving joy in this moment.

At an even deeper level of understanding, who are you if your body, mind and emotions change all the time? Is there a part of you that doesn't change? What new level of understanding can we bring to our lives knowing that everything changes? What becomes important? What becomes unimportant?

Summary of This Chapter

Playfulness

Emotional Intelligence

Going Within Yourself

Acceptance

Love

Using creativity and imagination – Express Yourself

Express Gratitude

Chapter 4

Are There Warning Signs of Suicide?

If depression is very serious and you're worried about people you care about than this chapter is a must read for you. These are warning signs that someone may be thinking about or planning to commit suicide include:

- They are always talking or thinking about death
- Clinical depression -- deep sadness, loss of interest, trouble sleeping and eating that gets worse
- Having a "death wish," tempting fate by taking risks that could lead to death, such as driving fast or running red lights
- Losing interest in things one used to care about
- Making comments about being hopeless, helpless, or worthless
- Putting affairs in order, tying up loose ends, changing a will
- Saying things like "it would be better if I wasn't here" or "I want out"
- Sudden, unexpected switch from being very sad to being very calm or appearing
- Talking about suicide or killing one's self

- Visiting or calling people to say goodbye

Where Can I Get Help for Suicide and Depression?

Encourage a suicidal or depressed person to seek the help of a mental health professional. Because the person may feel so hopeless that they may not think it's possible to be helped, you'll probably have to be persistent and go with that person.

If your loved one appears to be in imminent danger of committing suicide, do not leave him or her alone. Remove any weapons or drugs he or she could use. Accompany him or her to the nearest emergency room or call 911 (US). For other countries than US get informed for the right emergency number! NOW!

During treatment, be supportive. Help the person remember to take antidepressants or other prescribed medications and to continue any other therapy that's been prescribed.

Chapter 5.

How Can the Depression of Your Partner Affect Your Life?

From my experience.....

Your partner can't take over and for you this means more work certain obligations. On the other hand you get no recognition for helping the sick.

Many joint activities fall away and you lack common features that you have been connected to your partner. Your partner has no desire for sex, and more displays of affection.

He/she feels for you no more love and affection. He/she withdraws from the common friends, and possibly with him, so that you become isolated and feel lonely all the time.

Your partner threatens of suicide and you live in constant fear and stress.

Your partner is irritable and unapproachable and you feel rejected. Your commitment is **not** recognized.

Your partner makes no decisions and therefore you feel the responsibility for the family left alone. Your partner complains of physical problems on sleep or pain, and you are his constant complaints tired.

Your partner has difficulty concentrating, and you are annoyed when your partner makes mistakes. They are due to the constant complaints of your partner often irritable and run frequently from the skin.

This will be extremely hard period of your life. You might even want to leave your partner.

I wish you to stay strong!

Chapter 6

How to Respond to Your Partner's Depression

If you're like most families, you will toggle between different feelings and behaviors and forth.

You want to help your partner, but at the same time feel helpless and are not sure how to help him and how your help is taken from the patient. They want it back "as before" is, but see no way.

You use all your powers of persuasion and want to convince your partner that he sees everything black and there is hope for him.

They want to help, so that your partner quickly overcomes his depression. Therefore, you give him advice on what he can do, inform yourself fully aware of his illness and give him support.

You want to deliberately break your partner out of depression and make it again and again suggestions on what they could do together Beautiful. You might even suggest a holiday trip. But your partner makes a principle or may not also happy on vacation and you are disappointed.

1. You try to be strong and to have their own problems, but feel overwhelmed.

2. You should become an expert when it comes to depression, thankfully you're already reading this book.

3. You torture yourself with questions about what you can expect your partner or are, on what activities you are to exist, what work you need to remove it, etc.

4. You feel guilty to have done something wrong and to be responsible for your partner's depression.

5. You are a force, intentional and helpless because there is no improvement, and you do not know how to proceed.

6. You feel unfairly treated.

They are angry and short-tempered because when your partner no improvement in sight, and ask him to always energetic, he should get their act together.

They are annoying because everything only revolves around your partner.

You feel exploited and helpless because your partner times requested your help, sometimes rejects.

You feel with your worries not understood, must always be strong, while devolved the role of the needy.

You feel called into question and are angry because your partner does not answer your well-intentioned advice and nothing gets any better. As a result, you leave behind in your application.

You doubt your love and partnership.

Have you recognized in some of the feeling and reaction patterns? Sometimes condemn you for such thoughts and feelings?

All these thoughts and feelings are understandable and normal. If you accompany a depression sick partner for a long time, then consumed this also your mental and physical powers.

Chapter 7

Important to notice

Well-intentioned advice can often Depressive not accept or obey.

Physical contact in the form of petting or holding hands are usually experienced by depressed than pleasant.

Celebrations and social gatherings can strain the sick. The Council "You have to go under people" may be wrong and right, depending on which state of mind the depressive person is located.

There are phases in which the depressive feel even worse if it is among men. Amusement parks, funny movies or serene people reinforce usually the mental anguish of depressed because he has lost the ability to rejoice and to him, this is painfully aware of in such situations.

Think in everything you do and what your partner is doing depressive, mind: a depression is a mental disability. Because, these problems is through the eyes difficult to see, you can often only guess what is going on in your partner and what about him.

There may be ashamed of your partner to accept help. He/she feels it as a failure, and the other to admit that he needs help.

Make him/her repeatedly clear that there is no shame to seek help. After all, one goes also because of physical illness to the doctor.

Depression Help

Important Things to Remember

- Recognize the importance of the depression
- Do not underestimate your influence – <u>everything</u> matters
- Inform yourself about the topic of depression
- Motivate those who suffer from depression
- Do not overtax
- Pay close attention to word you choose
- Talk to friends and family
- Take suicidal thoughts seriously

40

Conclusion

"No bird soars too high if he soars with his own wings."

- William Blake

What if you have done all of the suggestions in this book and nothing is working? What if you still get up in the morning with that sense of dread or overwhelm? The truth is, some of us are in the wrong job, with the wrong partner, or living in the wrong part of the world. There may be elements of your life that just don't fit, that aren't right for you and that you do need to change. But here's the catch. You are not in the right place to take that on right now. You need to get a little better first before you take on those challenges from a more optimistic, hopeful and energized place. When you do get out of this season of depression, you will feel ready to take on new challenges and changes in your life. You'll be better equipped to do so. You'll have more emotional intelligence, energy, self-knowledge, innate happiness and well being, compassion and self-trust. This will all make you far more likely to succeed in bringing about the changes you deem necessary in your life.

We are never alone. Depression can be seen as a perfectly normal and natural part of life in today's world. It is a season in your life and seasons pass. We can find a way to enjoy and be grateful for all of our seasons.

None of these suggestions serve as a substitute for working with a professional. Seeing a therapist can be a great experience, helping you to reach your own understanding and insights in a safe and caring environment. If you want to see a professional, choose a therapist you feel you can open up to and trust. Don't hold back, go full out, but work at your own pace. Insights and healing come in their own time.

As your life changes, begin to use the understanding you have gained during your depression to live a whole-hearted, passion-led, playful and joyful life, and take any opportunity to help others suffering in depression by directing them to this book, or better yet, by being fully present with them and giving them your understanding, insight, compassion and encouragement.

Huge Thank You and Words of Gratitude!

First and foremost, Thank You for downloading this book. At the end of the day I'm **extremely** grateful for **every** download and **every** purchase. It really makes me smile and motivates me. I wish that every person would put their best forward for the human race. I wish you unlimited mental strength and discipline to achieve your goals and dreams. **Together** we can make the difference.

If you found the information useful I would be extremely grateful if you could write a short Amazon review. It really does make the difference and I personally read every review and take notes. I want to improve my books, so that I can provide more value to other people. I know that my future books will give you the best experience possible.

Download this book in Mp3 for FREE

I want to give you a little bonus for your purchase.

Please visit the following link for Audio Version.

http://eepurl.com/bsvBc9